ZACKBACK® SITTING

Other books by Dennis Zacharkow, PT

POSTURE: SITTING, STANDING, CHAIR DESIGN AND EXERCISE

WHEELCHAIR POSTURE AND PRESSURE SORES

ZACKBACK® SITTING

The Revolutionary Solution
for
Relieving Your Pain
and
Improving Your Posture!

Dennis Zacharkow, PT

ZACKBACK® International, Inc.
Rochester•Minnesota•USA

ZACKBACK® SITTING

ZACKBACK® is a registered trademark of ZACKBACK International, Inc.
VELCRO® is a registered trademark of theVelcro Companies
First Edition
ISBN: 0-9660169-3-9
Library of Congress Catalog Card Number: 97-61826

Published by ZACKBACK® International, Inc.
PO Box 9100
Rochester, MN 55903
Phone: 1-800-748-8464
FAX: 507-252-5150
Website: www.zackback.com

Cover design and illustrations by Gregory Wimmer
Printed in Canada by Hignell Printing Limited, Winnipeg, Manitoba

Publisher's Cataloging-in-Publication
(Provided by Quality Books, Inc.)

Zacharkow, Dennis.
    Zackback sitting : the revolutionary solution for relieving your pain and improving your posture! / Dennis Zacharkow. -- 1st ed.
    p. cm.
    Includes bibliographical references and index.
    Preassigned LCCN: 97-61826
    ISBN: 0-9660169-3-9

    1. Posture. 2. Backache--Prevention. 3. Carpal tunnel syndrome --Prevention. I. Title.

RA781.5.Z33 1998   613.7'8
                             QBI97-41363

ACKNOWLEDGMENTS

My thanks to the following individuals:

Vincent DelGobbo, Stephen Leale, Bruce Otis, Lori Redman, Frank Rocco, Steve Townsend, and Greg Znajda, PT, for reviewing the manuscript and for their valuable suggestions for improvement.

Gregory Wimmer for designing the cover and for his work on the line illustrations.

Jean Peterson for typing the manuscript.

Chris Young of Hignell Printing Limited for the special attention he gave to this project.

CONTENTS

PREFACE

Popular views on healthy sitting posture, such as the need for lumbar support and reclining backrests, are frequently based on concepts that are too fragmented in their approach to the human body. These views completely ignore how a change in alignment of one part of the body will alter the normal relationships between other parts of the body, and how this change in alignment will affect the body as a whole.

Many of these popular views, on closer examination, turn out to be misconceptions that have never been fully analyzed for their accuracy.

Why do these misconceptions continue to be accepted as correct by so many health professionals? Most likely because the health professions are not creative fields. They involve absorbing information in order to develop technical skills. As a result, many popular views are never questioned but are accepted as "fact."

With regard to sitting posture, the segmental approach to the human body has not always been the norm. In the late nineteenth and early twentieth centuries, schoolchildren's sitting posture was considered an area of extreme importance. Approached from a holistic rather than a segmental viewpoint, great emphasis was placed on the injurious effects improper seating had on breathing and on the development of postural deformities.

The encouraging news is that consumers are now taking a more active role in adopting healthier lifestyles. As more of us now sit for most of the day in front of a computer, understanding proper sitting posture is imperative for one's health. Therefore, I hope this book will inform you on how to achieve healthy, pain-free sitting for life.

Dennis Zacharkow

PART ONE

GENERAL SEATING ISSUES

Chapter 1

INTRODUCTION

The one activity that most of us do more than anything else throughout the day is **SIT!**

As the computer expands into more homes, businesses, and schools, improper sitting posture is becoming the major cause of lower back pain, upper back pain, neck pain, and carpal tunnel syndrome. Improper sitting posture is also a major cause of postural deformities such as round back and round shoulders.

Unfortunately, the above problems will continue to increase in our computer-driven information society. Why? — because the public has not received correct information from health professionals (M.D.s, physical therapists, chiropractors, ergonomists, etc.) and the office furniture industry regarding proper, healthy sitting posture!

Two of the most common misconceptions that have been enthusiastically advocated by health professionals and the office furniture industry for years are:

1. Lumbar support is the most important feature of a good chair to assure proper sitting posture.

The need for lumbar support is emphasized in almost every magazine and newspaper article listing important chair features, such as in the September 1996 issue of *Consumer Reports*.[1] A recent article in an occupational health and safety magazine was actually entitled

Lumbar Support Most Critical Feature To Consider During Chair Selection.[2]

2. Sitting upright is harmful; it is healthier to sit in a reclined position.

A 1995 *Wall Street Journal* article on sitting quotes a leading ergonomics expert as saying, "Don't sit up straight; Mother was never right about that."[3]

Another recent magazine article written by a specialist in office ergonomics states that ". . . a reclined backrest doesn't cause slouching; it improves posture."[4]

Besides these two specific misconceptions, a more general misconception is that **we are not designed to sit.**

This misconception was actually the first sentence of the previously mentioned *Wall Street Journal* article.[3] This would be an accurate statement if changed to read "We are not designed to sit *improperly.*"

As this book will show, there actually *is* an optimal healthy sitting posture which is extremely beneficial in the following ways:

- Relieving and preventing lower back pain, upper back pain, neck pain, shoulder pain, arm pain, wrist pain, hand pain, carpal tunnel syndrome, and thoracic outlet syndrome.

- Achieving proper use of your most important abdominal muscles for all of life's activities. (These important abdominal muscles are different from the

14

abdominal muscles exercised with the machines advertised on television.)

• Spontaneously achieving proper diaphragmatic breathing through stimulation to a key area of your back.

• Reducing your fatigue and increasing your productivity at work.

• Dramatically improving your posture and appearance, not only when sitting, but also when standing and walking.

• Preventing postural deformities from developing, such as round back and round shoulders.

However, before explaining the ZACKBACK Solution for achieving your optimal, pain-free, healthy sitting posture, let's explore the reasons why very few of us as adults sit as healthily as a nine-month-old infant!

Chapter 2

AN INFANT'S HEALTHY SITTING POSTURE — WHY WE LOSE IT

A nine-month-old infant can independently achieve and maintain a balanced, upright sitting posture with the proper upright relationship of the head, rib cage, and pelvis (Figure 1). As we grow up, there are three major factors in our society that result in the breakdown of our postural reflex mechanisms, the same postural reflex mechanisms that allow a nine-month-old infant to sit so well:

1. Improper backrest design of chairs.

Resting against the backrest of most chairs results in a distorted trunk posture, called a postural depression.[5] The term postural depression refers to a "hinging forward" of the front of the rib cage towards the pelvis. (Compare Figures 2-A and 2-B.) This postural depression also occurs when leaning forward improperly, and collapsing the weight of the trunk onto the arms (Figure 3).

Continually assuming a position of postural depression over the years will break down the normal postural reflex mechanism which involves proper activation of the abdominal muscles, back muscles, and diaphragm (the main breathing muscle).

2. Sitting at horizontal desks.

Using a horizontal desk for reading and writing forces one to bring the head forward to achieve the proper visual angle and visual distance to reading and writing materials. Continual use of horizontal desks alters the

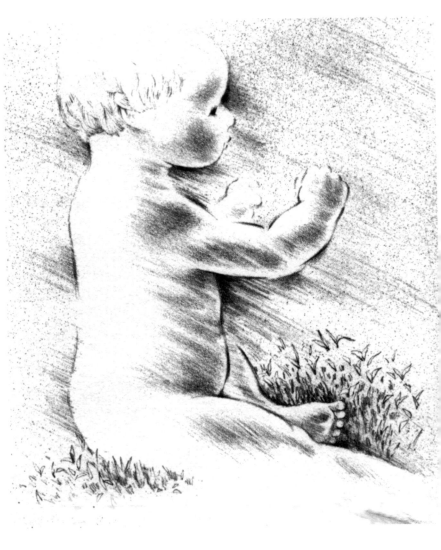

Figure 1.

Healthy sitting posture of a nine-month-old infant.

normal upright head-neck relationship, a key factor in proper body orientation.[6-9]

3. Heels on shoes.

Wearing heels on shoes results in a relaxation of important postural muscles of the foot. This causes a breakdown in the foot's postural reflex mechanism that is so critical for overall body posture.[10]

The typical low heel on the standard men's dress shoe decreases the normal tension (tone) of these postural muscles by about fifty percent. As the heel height on shoes increases to two inches and higher, there is a total relaxation of these critical postural muscles of the foot.[10]

Besides these three major cultural factors, the breakdown of our normal postural reflex mechanisms is intensified by several common sitting misconceptions.

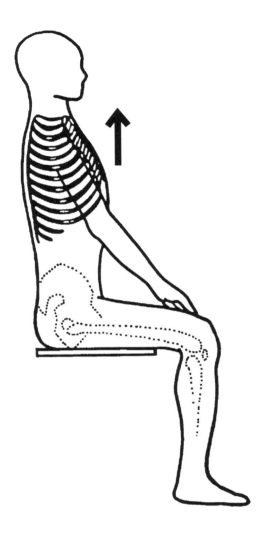

Figure 2-A.

Healthy upright sitting posture. Arrow refers to the elevated position of rib cage.

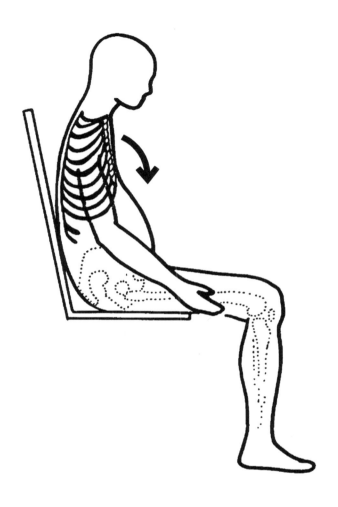

Figure 2-B.

Sitting in a postural depression. Arrow refers to "hinging forward" of rib cage towards the pelvis.

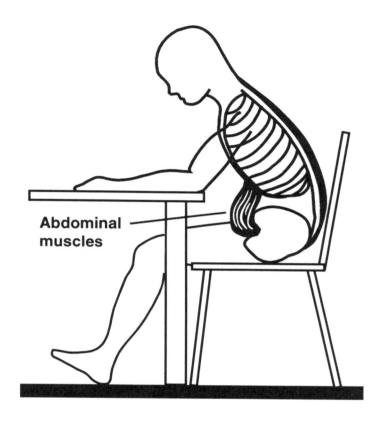

Abdominal muscles

Figure 3.

Postural depression due to improper forward leaning, with the weight of the trunk collapsed onto the arms. The abdominal muscles are relaxed, and there is a prolonged stretching of the back muscles and ligaments.

Chapter 3

COMMON
SITTING MISCONCEPTIONS

*"We have agreed to adjust our bodies to the dictates of chairs; only rarely do we find a chair that in its design has contracted to fulfill the requirements of the human body. In such ways have we permitted the forms and products of our culture to change our body alignments in order to satisfy **their** structural requirements. We have accustomed ourselves to habitual modes of use that are literally disfiguring"* (Leibowitz, 1967).[11]

LUMBAR SUPPORT

If not from one's own personal experience, most people know someone who has been to a doctor, physical therapist, or chiropractor and was given a large foam roll or cushion (called a lumbar support) to use behind the lower back when sitting (Figure 4). The intended purpose for the lumbar support is to maintain the lumbar lordosis, the curve in the lower back that is normally present in the *standing* position.

The Problems With Lumbar Support

1. The first problem with lumbar support, and why the use of lumbar supports is a fallacy, is that there is a

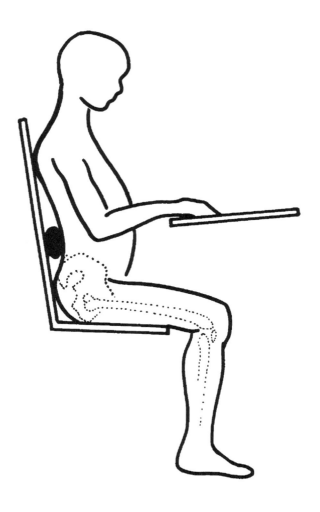

Figure 4.

Sitting with lumbar support. Note the unhealthy backwards displacement of the upper trunk, and the overstretching of the abdominal muscles.

natural flattening of the curve in the lower back when going from a standing to a sitting position (Figure 5).[12-14]

2. The second problem with lumbar support is that it distorts the proper upright relationship of the rib cage and pelvis, with the upper trunk being displaced behind the hips.[15,16] (See Figure 4.) This backwards displacement of the upper trunk with lumbar support moves one further away from his/her work surface (desk, keyboard, steering wheel of car). Trying to maintain this sitting posture when working often causes increased stress to the neck and upper back.

3. The third problem with lumbar support is that no lumbar support is possible in a forward-leaning posture, which is a very common working position. Once you lean forward from the backrest, lumbar support cannot be used.[15,16]

4. The fourth problem with lumbar support is that it results in a relaxation and overstretching of the abdominal muscles, which are critical postural muscles for both sitting and standing posture.[15,16]

RECLINING BACKRESTS

According to the *Wall Street Journal* article mentioned in the introduction, "In offices, modestly reclining office chairs are in vogue today."[3] The same article quotes a group product manager at a major office furniture manufacturer as predicting that for future working postures, "we'll be lying down 10 years from now, maybe."[3]

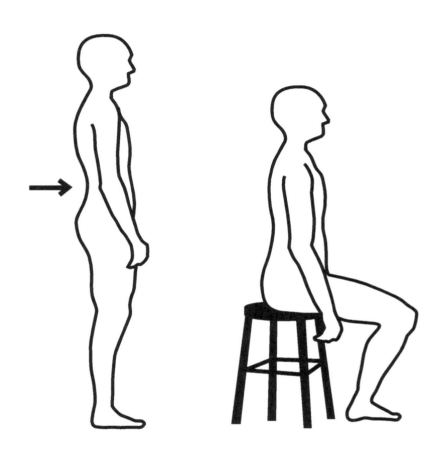

Figure 5.

Arrow refers to the curve in the lower back when standing. There is
a natural flattening of this curve when going from standing to sitting.

If the goal is total atrophy of the back and abdominal muscles, modestly to extremely reclined trunk postures when sitting would have some validity!

This embracing of the concept of reclined work postures by many health professionals and members of the office furniture industry shows a total misunderstanding of the proper functioning of the human body.

The Problems with Reclining Backrests

1. A reclining backrest distorts the proper upright relationship of the head, neck, and upper back. This is because when working at a computer or desk (similar to driving an automobile), the visual requirements of the task are critical.

In order to achieve the proper visual angle and distance to the computer screen, desk, or the windshield of a car while in a reclined posture, one will pull the head, neck, and upper back forward and out of vertical alignment (Figure 6).

Besides distorting the proper head/neck/upper back relationship, this reclined posture increases the potential for neck pain, upper back pain, and headaches.

2. Reclining results in a position of postural depression, with relaxation of the abdominal and back muscles, along with poor diaphragmatic breathing.

When sitting in a moderately to extremely reclined posture, one has the same trunk muscle activity as an unconscious person!

3. The greater the recline to the backrest at the computer or in the car, the more the arms must extend

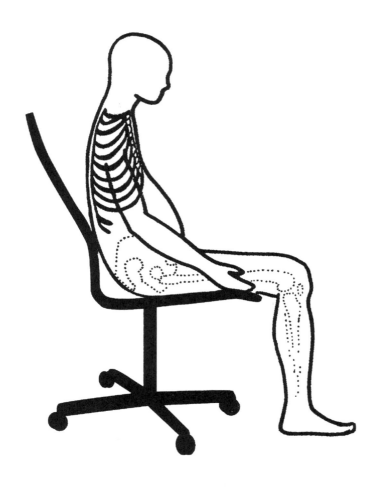

Figure 6.

When sitting in a reclined posture, one will pull the head, neck, and upper back forward to achieve proper vision for the task being performed.

forward in order to reach the keyboard or steering wheel. This increases the stress to the neck, shoulder, and upper back muscles when typing or driving.

4. Reclining distorts the proper upright relationship of the trunk and pelvis, by positioning the trunk behind the pelvis (Figure 7). The result is a marked distortion in body alignment, yet this posture is considered normal! However, who would consider it "normal" if observing someone standing or walking with their trunk positioned behind the pelvis (Figure 8)?

WHAT THE POPULAR MISCONCEPTIONS OF LUMBAR SUPPORT AND RECLINING BACKRESTS IGNORE

By ignoring a holistic approach to analyzing optimal healthy sitting posture, the proponents of lumbar support and reclining backrests dismiss many important seating issues such as sitting stability, proper alignment of the thoracic spine, and proper respiration.

Key Areas of Instability When Sitting

Pelvis

Compared to standing where the hip joints are close to a fully extended (straightened) position, the hip joints are in a mid-position when sitting. This results in the freedom of the pelvis to "rock" or "oscillate" over the sitting bones, called the ischial tuberosities (Figure 9).[17]

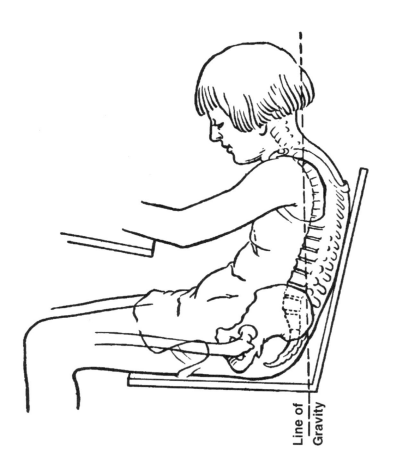

Line of
Gravity

Figure 7.

Notice how the trunk is positioned behind the pelvis in a reclined
sitting posture. From Bennett, H.E.: *School Posture and Seating.*
Boston, Ginn and Company, 1928.

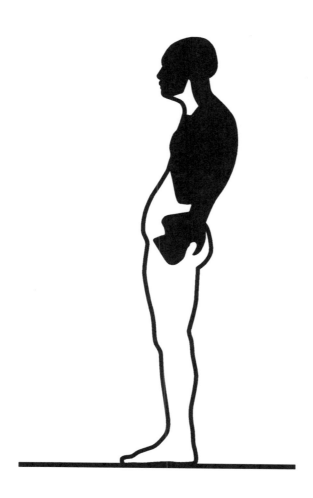

Figure 8.

Would anyone consider this to be a normal standing posture, with the trunk positioned behind the pelvis? This same trunk posture, however, is considered quite normal when sitting! From McKenzie, R.T.: *Exercise in Education and Medicine*, 2nd ed. Philadelphia, Saunders, 1915.

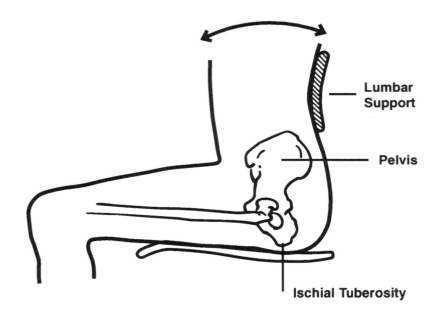

Figure 9.

Side view of the pelvis and hip joint when sitting. Arrows refer to the oscillatory movements of the pelvis rocking over the ischial tuberosities. Notice how lumbar support is placed too high to control this movement of the pelvis. Adapted from Bennett, H.E.: *School Posture and Seating.* Boston, Ginn and Company, 1928.

The rocking motion of the pelvis over the ischial tuberosities when sitting is a major cause of stress to the lower back.[18] Lumbar support completely ignores this pelvic instability, as lumbar support is prescribed to be placed just above the pelvis.[19]

Rib Cage

The rib cage is the second key area of instability ignored by proponents of lumbar support and reclining backrests. When leaning back against the typical reclined backrest, the rib cage hinges forward towards the pelvis in a position of postural depression (Figure 10). A similar hinging forward of the rib cage towards the pelvis is found in typical upright and forward-leaning postures (Figure 11).

The rib cage hinges forward towards the pelvis due to the spine flexing in an area just above the lower back, called the **lower thoracic spine**[20-25] (Figure 12). More specifically, this "hinge area" for spinal flexion involves the tenth thoracic vertebra through the twelfth thoracic vertebra (T10-T12). Lumbar support does not stabilize this critical area of the spine.

The lower thoracic spine is where the greatest degree of spinal flexion occurs with improper sitting postures. The hinging forward of the rib cage towards the pelvis when sitting, through flexion of the lower thoracic spine, is similar to the hinging forward that occurs with sit-up exercises and toe-touching exercises.

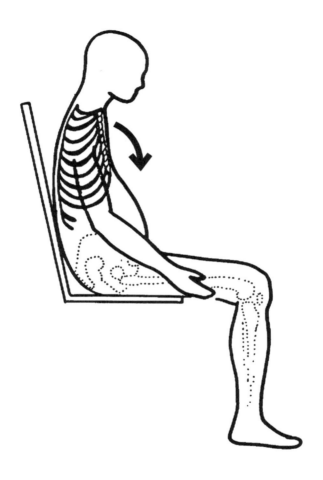

Figure 10.

Postural depression in a reclined sitting posture. Arrow refers to hinging forward of the rib cage towards the pelvis.

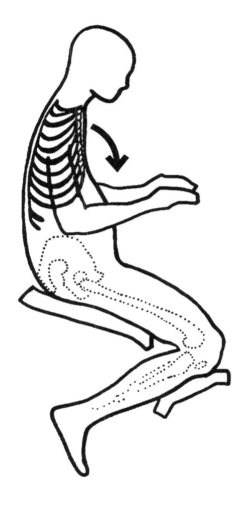

Figure 11.

Postural depression in an upright sitting posture on a kneeling chair. Arrow refers to hinging forward of the rib cage towards the pelvis.

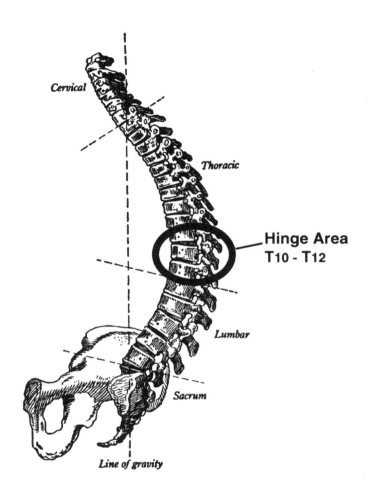

Figure 12.

Circle denotes area of the thoracic spine responsible for the hinging forward of the rib cage towards the pelvis. Adapted from Bennett, H.E.: *School Posture and Seating*. Boston, Ginn and Company, 1928.

NOTE: Although not shown here, the "hinge area" for spinal flexion also includes L1, the uppermost lumbar vertebra.

By rotating Figure 13-A ninety degrees clockwise, this classic illustration from 1899 shows how the postural depression resulting from sit-up exercises and "crunches" (Figure 13-B) is very similar to the postural depression in common sitting postures (Figure 13-A).

Other Issues Ignored

By focusing solely on lumbar support or a reclining backrest, an important postural principle expressed by Haynes in 1928 is ignored: "The position and use of each part of the body must be considered in relation to all the other parts, for that which affects one part directly affects all the other parts indirectly."[26]

For example, the popular simplistic solution of a reclining backrest distorts the proper upright relationship of the head, neck, upper back, rib cage, and pelvis. The effect of reclining the trunk also results in a relaxation of the abdominal muscles, leading to an impairment of proper diaphragmatic breathing.

Therefore, a holistic approach to optimal healthy sitting posture must address the following issues:

1. Proper stabilization of the pelvis and rib cage.
2. Proper diaphragmatic breathing.
3. Proper upright relationship of the head, rib cage, and pelvis.
4. Proper use of the abdominal muscles.
5. Proper trunk stabilization to allow free movement of the arms when working, as opposed to collapsing the weight of the trunk through the arms and onto the desk, armrests of the chair, or wrist rest of the keyboard.

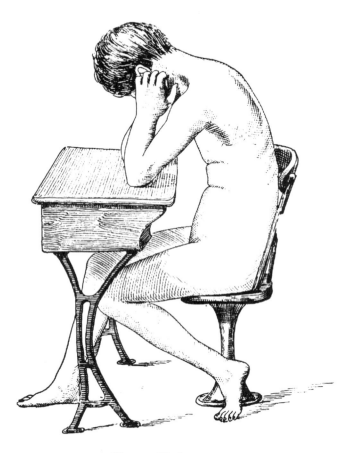

Figure 13-A.

Notice how the postural depression when sitting (A) is similar to the postural depression resulting from sit-up exercises and "crunches" (B). From Bradford, E.H., and Stone, J.S.: The seating of school children. *Transactions of the American Orthopedic Association*, *12*:170-183, 1899.

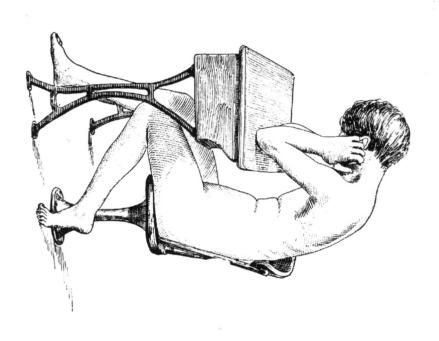

Figure 13-B.

PART TWO

SPECIFIC SEATING ISSUES

Chapter 4

BREATHING

One of the most important issues to address in healthy sitting posture is also the most ignored: proper diaphragmatic breathing.

Proper diaphragmatic breathing involves a raised position of the diaphragm at the start of inspiration due to proper activation of the abdominal muscles (Figure 14-A). This abdominal muscle activity continues throughout inspiration.[27,28] (Ask any opera singer.) Proper activation of the abdominal muscles also improves the diaphragm's ability to lift the lower ribs, and hence to expand the lower rib cage.

However, when sitting in a position of postural depression, with the rib cage hinging forward towards the pelvis, there is a relaxation of the abdominal muscles and a lowered position of the diaphragm at the start of inspiration (Figure 14-B). This sitting posture not only restricts diaphragmatic breathing, it also facilitates unhealthy upper chest breathing.

Upper chest breathing increases the respiratory load placed on the scalene muscles, the neck muscles attached to the upper two ribs (Figure 15). The scalene muscles normally contribute to inspiration through elevation of the upper two ribs. However, when upper chest breathing predominates, the scalene muscles are overworked.

The tendency for the rib cage to move in a downward direction when sitting in a position of postural

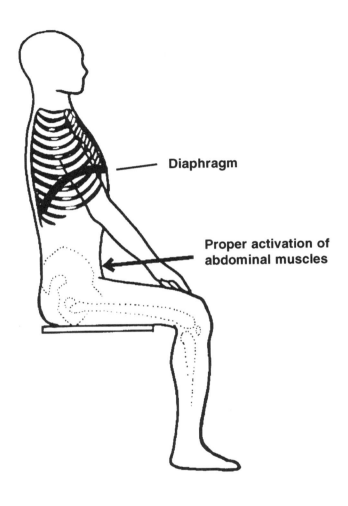

Figure 14-A.

Healthy sitting posture involves a raised position of the diaphragm due to proper activation of the abdominal muscles. Note in particular the greater depth and expansion of the lower rib cage.

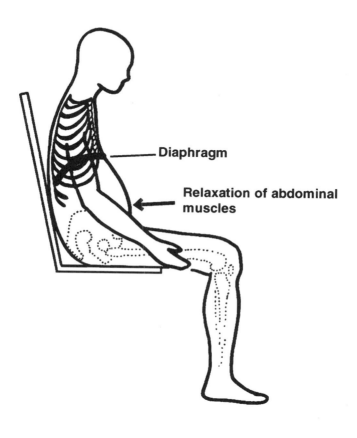

Figure 14-B.

When sitting in a postural depression, there is a relaxation of the
abdominal muscles and a lowered position of the diaphragm.
Diaphragmatic breathing will be restricted and upper chest
breathing will be emphasized.

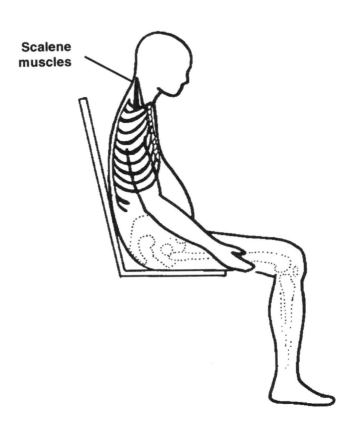

Scalene muscles

Figure 15.

Sitting in a postural depression will restrict diaphragmatic breathing and result in overuse of the scalene muscles through upper chest breathing.

depression also results in a greater load on the scalene muscles to elevate the upper rib cage against gravity.[29,30]

The bad news here is that overuse of the scalene muscles not only strains the neck, but may also activate "trigger points" in these muscles. These trigger points can result in pain down the arms and hands that is similar to the pain pattern of carpal tunnel syndrome.[31]

More bad news is that shortening of the scalene muscles from overuse in upper chest breathing and stabilizing the rib cage may compress nerves and blood vessels in the lower neck/upper chest region. This is called thoracic outlet syndrome, which frequently occurs in association with carpal tunnel syndrome but is often not diagnosed.[32-35]

The good news is that the ZACKBACK Solution prevents overuse of the scalene muscles by providing mechanical support to stabilize the rib cage.

More good news is that the ZACKBACK Solution also prevents overuse of the scalene muscles by facilitating proper diaphragmatic breathing. This activation of the diaphragm occurs through reflexes that are elicited by isolated pressure stimulation to the lower thoracic region of the back.[36,37] (These reflexes are discussed further in Chapter 10.)

Chapter 5

THE ABDOMINAL MUSCLES

Most abdominal exercises such as sit-ups and "crunches" primarily strengthen the upper portion of the rectus abdominis, the most superficial and vertical abdominal muscle[38-40] (Figure 16). These exercises actually reinforce a sitting and standing postural depression, by pulling the rib cage forward and down.[21]

In addition, when most individuals attempt to flatten their stomachs, they constrict the upper abdomen by improperly contracting the upper portion of the rectus abdominis. The resulting posture interferes with proper functioning of the diaphragm and actually weakens the lower abdominal region.[41,42]

The most important abdominal muscle for healthy sitting and standing is not the rectus, but the transversus abdominis, the deepest abdominal muscle. Unlike the rectus, the transversus muscle fibers run horizontally, and therefore cannot pull the rib cage towards the pelvis (Figure 17).

The transversus is the critical abdominal muscle for proper diaphragmatic breathing. It is also the critical abdominal muscle for increasing intra-abdominal pressure, thereby "elongating" the lumbar spine and reducing stress on the lower back (Figure 18).[43,44] (Another muscle that works with the transversus abdominis for increasing intra-abdominal pressure is the lower part of the internal oblique abdominal muscle.[44,45] Similar to the transversus, these muscle fibers also run in a horizontal direction.)

49

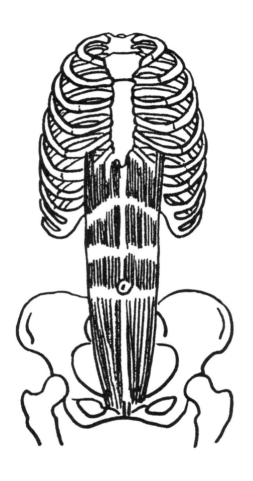

Figure 16.

The rectus abdominis muscle. Sit-ups and "crunches" primarily
strengthen the upper rectus, the part of the muscle
above the belly button.

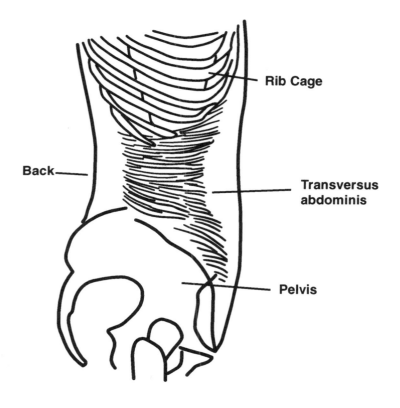

Rib Cage

Back

Transversus
abdominis

Pelvis

Figure 17.

The right transversus abdominis muscle. Note the horizontal
direction of the muscle fibers.

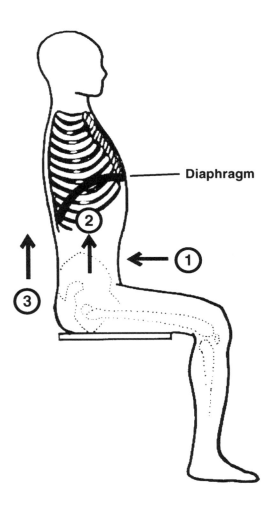

Diaphragm

Figure 18.

Proper activation of the transversus abdominis muscle (1) will raise
the intra-abdominal pressure (2) for proper, healthy sitting posture.
The result will be an "elongating" of the lumbar spine (3), thereby
reducing the compressive stress on the lower back.

A recent study in the journal *Spine* has shown how critical the transversus muscle is in providing proper trunk stabilization for arm movement.[46] In this study, the transversus was the only trunk muscle that contracted before the contraction of the shoulder muscles in raising the upper arm forwards. Interestingly, in individuals with low back pain, contraction of the transversus was delayed until after contraction of the shoulder muscles. This indicates a breakdown of the trunk stabilization mechanism in individuals with low back pain.

In summary, the bad news is that sit-ups, "crunches," and abdominal machine workouts will reinforce a position of postural depression.

The good news is that with the ZACKBACK Solution, one can easily achieve proper activation of the critical transversus muscle when sitting, which is easily carried over into standing and other postures and movements.

Chapter 6

ARMRESTS

In all animals other than humans, the shoulders and arms serve to support the trunk. However, with our upright posture on two feet, the arms are no longer required to support the trunk. Instead, a postural reflex mechanism of the trunk muscles has evolved to provide stabilization for independent arm movement.[47]

Unfortunately, from constant sitting in a position of postural depression, this postural reflex mechanism of trunk stabilization has broken down. As can be observed at most computer workstations, human posture has actually reverted to that of the animal kingdom, with the arms functioning to support the collapsed trunk! This is accomplished by weight bearing heavily on the armrests of the chair, the front edge of the desk, or the wrist rest of the keyboard (Figure 19).

The bad news here is that the increased weight bearing on a wrist rest in these frequently observed postures increases the pressure directly over the carpal tunnel region and the underlying median nerve, thereby increasing the risk of developing carpal tunnel syndrome.

In addition, armrests and wrist rests should *not* be used when operating the keyboard. The reason is that armrest and wrist rest use eliminates the participation of all muscle groups above elbow level in the keying movement.[48] The resulting increased workload placed on the

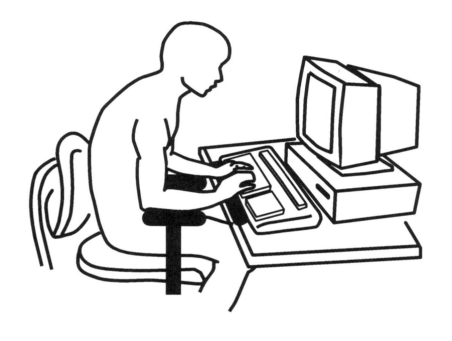

Figure 19.

Human posture has reverted to that of the animal kingdom, with the arms functioning to support the collapsed trunk.

forearms and hands may lead to muscle damage and tendinitis characteristic of cumulative trauma disorders.[49]

Proper keyboard operation involves using the entire upper extremities, starting at the shoulder joints, in a slight forwards and backwards gliding motion over the keys. This is accomplished *without* any arm or wrist support. Proper movement of the mouse and other pointing devices also involves using the entire upper extremity, with the upper arm kept close to the side of the body.[50] In tasks where mouse use predominates over keyboard use, the keyboard should be placed off center, and the mouse should be given the prominent position in front of the body.

The good news here is that the ZACKBACK Solution with proper activation of the abdominals (transversus abdominis) and proper support to the lower thoracic spine to stabilize the rib cage, facilitates proper keyboard and mouse operation *without arm support!*

Proper unsupported arm posture at the keyboard is with the upper arms vertical and the forearms slightly below horizontal[51,52] (Figure 20). Compared to keeping the forearms either horizontal or above horizontal, a downward slope of the forearms (slightly below horizontal) reduces the stress to the neck and upper back.[53]

The downward slope of the forearms will also facilitate maintaining a healthy, straight wrist posture when typing.[54,55] This is important for reducing the risk of developing carpal tunnel syndrome.

Another frequent site of nerve compression with keyboard operation is the elbow region, involving the ulnar nerve. This is called cubital tunnel syndrome. A downward slope of the forearm, along with keeping the

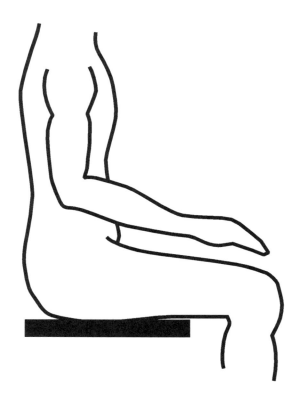

Figure 20.

Proper unsupported arm posture at the keyboard is with the upper arms vertical and the forearms slightly below horizontal.

upper arm vertical and the wrist straight, will reduce the stress on the ulnar nerve.[56]

Therefore, proper keyboard height with a downward slope of the forearms will be just above the thighs, a position much lower than traditionally advocated. The keyboard or keyboard tray should have a slight downward slope (approximately 10 degrees) to match the downward slope of the forearms[57] (Figure 21).

> **Important Note:** If you need to look *frequently* at the keyboard for feedback when typing, this lowered keyboard position may increase the stress to your neck and upper back.[54] The best compromise will then be a slightly higher keyboard and forearm position.

Although armrests on a chair should not be used when typing, they do have other important functions:

1. They reduce stress to the hips, knees, and back when getting in and out of the chair.

2. They provide intermittent support when taking rest breaks from typing.

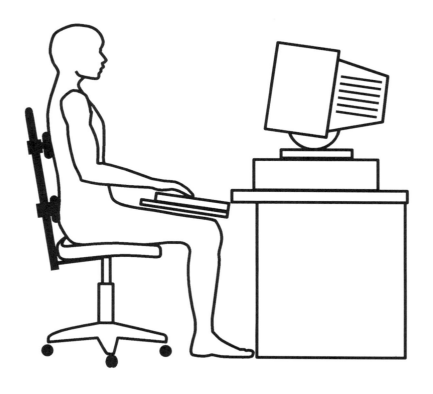

Figure 21.

Proper keyboard posture, with a slight downward slope to
the keyboard or keyboard tray to match the downward slope
of the forearms.

Chapter 7

ROUND SHOULDERS

"Pull your shoulders back!" Most of us have heard that command at one time or another from a teacher, therapist, or parent.

Strengthening the muscles between the shoulder blades to correct a round shoulders posture is an example of a segmental approach to posture that is also a misconception. A physical therapy study in 1990 did not support the prescription of muscle strengthening exercises to correct a round shoulders posture.[58]

A holistic approach to posture considers round shoulders to be a general disturbance of the body's balance.[59] In the sitting position, lower thoracic spinal posture, pelvic posture, head posture, and arm posture are all interrelated to round shoulders (Figure 22).

Therefore, round shoulders result from flexion of the lower thoracic spine, excessive forward or backward tilting of the pelvis, a reaching forward of the head, and a raising forward of the upper arms from their balanced vertical position at the sides of the hips.[60,61]

So, the bad news is that pulling the shoulders back when sitting will not correct a round shoulders posture. Moreover, it will only result in a different postural deviation that distorts proper body alignment and fatigues the upper back!

The good news is that by correcting the postural depression, or forward hinging of the rib cage towards the pelvis, the ZACKBACK Solution restores the proper

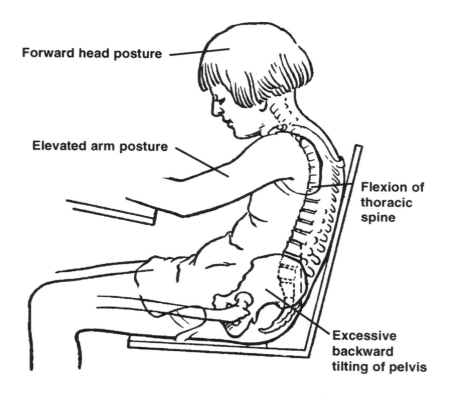

Forward head posture

Elevated arm posture

Flexion of thoracic spine

Excessive backward tilting of pelvis

Figure 22.

Round shoulders is a general disturbance of the body's balance, involving lower thoracic spinal posture, head posture, pelvic posture, and arm posture. Adapted from Bennett, H.E.: *School Posture and Seating*. Boston, Ginn and Company, 1928.

alignment of the shoulders. As long as pressure is maintained against the support to the lower thoracic spine (positioned just below the shoulder blades), the shoulders will be in proper alignment. (Proper ZACKBACK support is discussed in detail in Chapter 10.)

Round shoulders is an important seating issue, because the resulting distorted posture is a major factor in the development of thoracic outlet syndrome.[61,62] (See Chapter 4.)

Chapter 8

THE SEAT SURFACE

Two areas of the body that have evolved to withstand great external pressures are the heels of the feet and the sitting bones (ischial tuberosities). The ischial tuberosities are the most important areas for weight bearing on the seat, as they provide the important reference points for coordinated movement of the trunk and limbs.[63,64] They are the pivot points for shifting the trunk forwards and backwards. A secondary region for weight bearing on the seat is the upper half of the back of the thighs.[65]

Three areas *not* suitable for weight bearing on the seat are (Figure 23):

1. The tail bone (coccyx). Weight bearing on the tail bone occurs when sitting on a soft seat, or when sitting in a position of postural depression, especially with a reclined backrest.

2. The bony projections adjacent to the hip joints (greater trochanters of the femurs). Based on their structure and function, the trochanters are completely unsuited for supporting the body weight in a sitting position.[66] Try sitting for an extended period of time in a car with an extreme bucket seat, or better yet on a toilet seat!

3. The back of the lower thighs, just behind the knees. Pressure in this region of the thighs obstructs venous blood flow from the lower legs, resulting in lower leg swelling and discomfort.

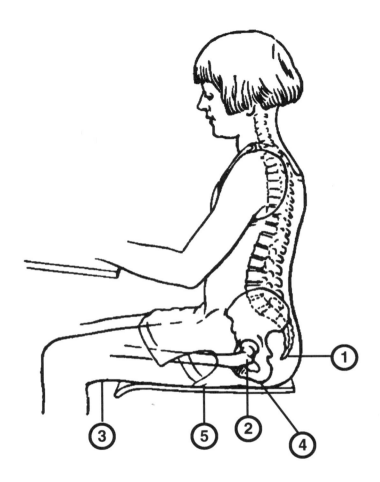

Figure 23.

Areas of the body not suitable for weight bearing on the seat are the tail bone (1), the bony projections adjacent to the hip joints (2), and the back of the lower thighs (3). The two major weight bearing areas should be the ischial tuberosities (4) and the upper half of the back of the thighs (5). Adapted from Bennett, H.E.: *School Posture and Seating*. Boston, Ginn and Company, 1928.

IMPORTANT SEAT FEATURES FOR PROPER STABILIZATION

Seat Upholstery

The seat upholstery should be firm, rather than soft, in order to properly stabilize the pelvis. With soft cushioning, an increase in muscle activity is necessary to stabilize the sitter.

Seat Fabric

The seat fabric should have sufficient surface friction (such as a woven fabric) to prevent sliding forward on the seat, and losing contact with the lower backrest.

Bad news: Expensive leather office chairs and car seats will cause you to sit in a postural depression.

Good news: You save money and sit better on a woven fabric!

Seat Height

The most stable sitting posture is with the feet firmly on the floor. Therefore, an adjustable seat height on a chair is essential. A footrest is necessary if the seat height does not lower sufficiently, or if one's desk is too high. (A height-adjustable desk and separate height-adjustable keyboard surface are critical workstation components to assure a proper working posture.)

Seat Depth

There should be at least 1-2 inches of clearance between the front edge of the seat and the back of the knees. If the seat depth is too long, there is difficulty maintaining contact with the lower backrest.

Seat Slope

In order to maintain proper stabilization against the lower part of the backrest, there should be a slight backward slope (approximately 5 degrees) to the seat surface. Therefore, the knees will be positioned slightly higher than the hips when sitting. (See Figure 23.)

A popular trend in seating over the last two decades has been a forward-sloping seat, where the knees are positioned lower than the hips (Figure 24). Contrary to the claims that forward-sloping seats will improve one's sitting posture, these chair designs actually destabilize the body and cause the pelvis to slide forward on the seat. An increase in leg muscle activity is then necessary to counteract this forward thrust on the seat.

Due to the forward displacement of the center of gravity with a forward-sloping seat, the individual will eventually slump forward and achieve trunk stabilization by leaning heavily on the armrests of the chair, the front edge of the desk, or the wrist rest of the keyboard.[67]

A Scandinavian study investigating forward- and backward-sloping seats found a tendency for less foot swelling with backward-sloping seats.[68] The same study also found the beneficial pressure exerted against the

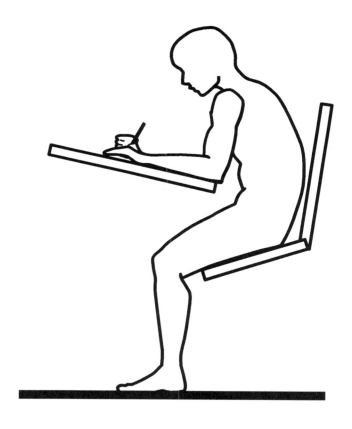

Figure 24.

A forward-sloping seat will destabilize the body and cause the pelvis to slide forward on the seat. The end result will be a postural depression, with the arms functioning to support the collapsed trunk.

backrest to be twice as high with a backward-sloping seat compared to a forward-sloping seat.

Chapter 9

HEAD POSTURE AND VISION

As early as 1865, Dr. Fahrner of Zurich, Switzerland stressed an important postural principle that is just as critical today: The first slight reaching forward of the head is the start of the postural collapse when sitting.[60]

This slight forward bend of the head, a major cause of neck pain, back pain, and headaches, is due to reading and writing at horizontal desks, and gazing at computer screens that are positioned too low. Why does a horizontal desk for reading and writing or a low computer screen height result in the head being brought forward from its balanced, upright posture? Simply because the line of sight must be perpendicular to the book, paper, or screen in order to see it clearly (Figure 25).

(With computer work, there may be a slight trade-off regarding the line of sight being perpendicular to the screen. It may be necessary to tilt the screen downwards to avoid glare.)

READING POSTURE

The correct position for reading while maintaining an upright head posture is with the book perpendicular to the line of sight, approximately 60 degrees from the horizontal, 14-20 inches from the eyes (depending on the print, light, and the eyes of the reader), and approximately at the height of the chin.[65]

Proper reading posture can be accomplished with an adjustable reading stand (Figure 26).

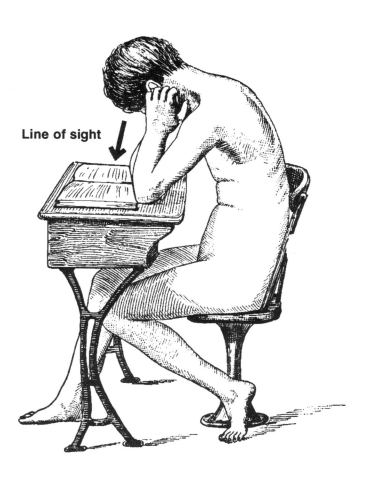

Line of sight

Figure 25.

The head will always be brought forward from its balanced, upright posture at a horizontal desk in order to facilitate vision.
From Bradford, E.H. and Stone, J.S.: The seating of school children. *Transactions of the American Orthopaedic Association, 12*:170-183, 1899.

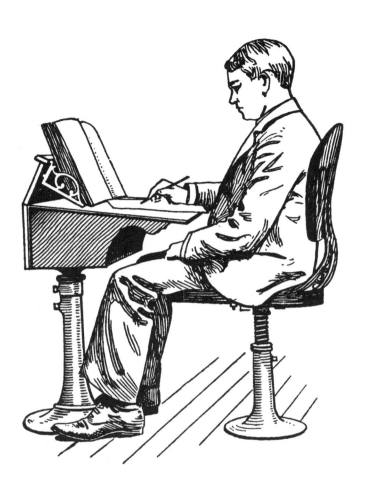

Figure 26.

Reading stands such as the one illustrated here were very common in schools during the late 1800s and early 1900s. Over the last decade, several models of portable, adjustable reading stands have become available. From Mosher, E.M.: Hygienic desks for school children. *Educational Review, 18*:9-14, June 1899.

WRITING POSTURE

Writing at a desk with a high inclination may cause books, papers, and pens to slide off the desk, and it may also lead to an increase in arm fatigue. Therefore, the best compromise for a writing surface is an inclination of 10 to 15 degrees from the horizontal, keeping the upper arm vertical, and the forearm inclined from the horizontal to coincide with the plane of the desk top inclination[69] (Figure 27).

This inclination for writing can be accomplished on many desks by slightly elevating the two desk legs located furthest from the chair. The slightly inclined writing surface can then be enhanced with an adjustable reading stand for proper reading posture.

COMPUTER POSTURE

Regarding computer work, the further one can sit from the screen, the better, as it is more relaxing for the eyes and reduces fatigue.[70] This is why a large computer screen with greater height to the characters is recommended.[70]

The recommended viewing distance for current computer screens is approximately 25 to 40 inches from the eyes to the screen.[71,72] To maintain an upright head posture with the eyes naturally directed slightly downward, the center of the computer screen should be positioned approximately 10 to 15 degrees below eye level (Figure 28).

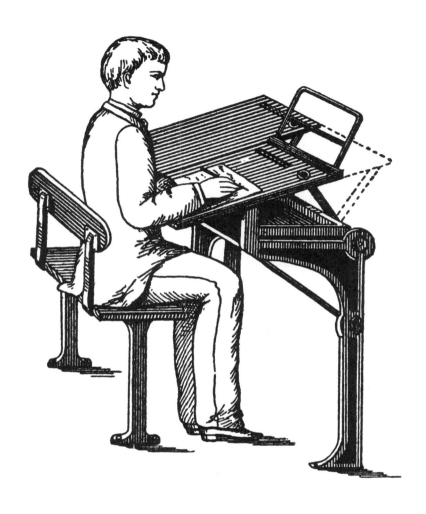

Figure 27.

Proper writing posture, with the upper arm vertical and the forearm
inclined from the horizontal to coincide with the plane of the desk
top inclination. From Burgerstein, L. and Netolitzky, A.: *Handbuch
der Schulhygiene.* Jena, Verlag Von Gustav Fischer, 1895.

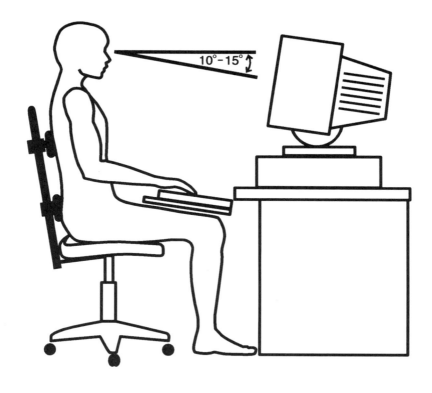

Figure 28.

To maintain an upright head posture, the viewing angle to the center of the computer screen should be approximately 10 to 15 degrees. (The viewing angle is the angle formed by a horizontal line at eye level with the line connecting the eye and the center of the screen.)

When one's work involves viewing both the computer screen and paper documents, traditional ergonomic guidelines recommend placing both the screen and documents at the same viewing distance from the eyes (approximately 20 inches). This identical viewing distance is considered necessary to prevent eye fatigue. However, contrary to expectation, eye fatigue does not increase when the computer screen is placed at a greater viewing distance from the eyes than the paper documents.[73,74] Therefore, the document and screen viewing distances should each be determined based on one's comfort.

Bifocals

Bifocal wearers are at special risk for developing neck pain, back pain, and headaches from viewing the computer screen. The bottom portion of the bifocal lens is commonly designed for a 16 inch viewing distance and a downward viewing angle of approximately 25 degrees. As the computer screen is located further away (25 to 40 inches) and higher in the viewing field (a downward viewing angle of 10 to 15 degrees), the bifocal wearer ends up tilting the head back and leaning forward towards the computer screen.[75,76]

Bifocal users should consult with an eye doctor knowledgeable in computer visual problems for a more appropriate prescription and lens design.

PART THREE

HEALTHY, PAIN-FREE SITTING

Chapter 10

THE ZACKBACK SOLUTION

The ZACKBACK Solution for healthy, pain-free sitting involves a unique supporting system for the pelvis and the rib cage. These are the two critical areas requiring stabilization that are neglected by both the lumbar support and reclining backrest concepts.

SACRAL SUPPORT

The key to stabilizing the pelvis in its proper neutral position (mid-position) is to provide support to the area just below the lumbar spine (lower back) called the sacrum (Figure 29). The sacroiliac joints, the joints connecting the sacrum to the pelvis that are a common site for low back pain, are also stabilized with the ZACKBACK Solution. (See Figure 29.)

If the pelvis is tilted forward from its proper neutral position, there is a spontaneous relaxation and over-stretching of the abdominal muscles. If the pelvis is tilted too far backward, the spine flexes and the tail bone bears weight on the seat. Therefore, *do not* actively arch your lower back when being fitted for sacral support. Sit in a relaxed, upright posture.

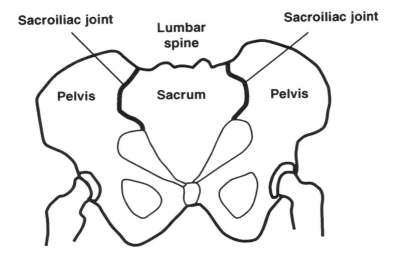

Figure 29.

The sacrum is located just below the lumbar spine (lower back).
The sacroiliac joints connect the sacrum to each side of the pelvis.

Location of Sacral Support

To find the proper location for sacral support, locate the right and left upper edges of your pelvis (Figure 30). To find the upper edges of your pelvis, place your thumbs on your belly button. Then slide each thumb directly sideways in opposite directions until the thumbs are at the sides of your waist. Now, if you lower your thumbs no more than approximately 1 inch from this position, you should feel the upper edges of your pelvis.

Based on comfort, the upper border of the sacral support should be positioned approximately 1 to 2 inches below the upper edges of your pelvis. (See Figure 30.) For a mock-up sacral support, attach to your chair in the proper location using VELCRO® or tape, a firm piece of foam approximately 4 inches in height, 10 inches wide, and 1 inch thick.

Important Note: The proper seat height is critical for maintaining firm contact with the sacral support. The feet should be firmly on the floor (or a footrest), with the weight bearing on the seat over the sitting bones (ischial tuberosities) and the upper half of the back of the thighs. (Refer to Chapter 8 and Figure 23.) If the seat is too high, the pelvis will slide forward on the seat, and you will lose contact with the sacral support.

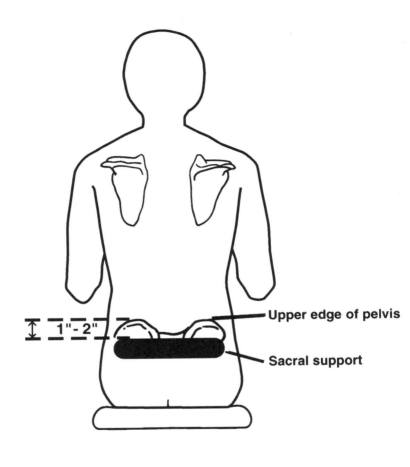

Figure 30.

Proper location of sacral support.

How to Activate Your Abdominal Muscles When Sitting

With the sacral support in position, it is easy to learn how to activate your critical abdominal muscle, the transversus abdominis.

Without holding your breath or straining, concentrate on gently pressing back against the sacral support in a backward and upward direction (Figure 31). At first, it is natural for this movement to result in an overflow of activity to other muscles that also lengthen the body, such as the quadriceps (front thigh muscles) and the soleus (calf muscles).

With practice, this leg muscle activity will be eliminated, resulting in just a slight backward movement of the pelvis and a "belly-in" position of the lower abdomen, due to contraction of the lower transversus abdominis and the lower internal oblique abdominal muscle.[77-79] When done properly, this movement does not interfere with respiration, and it does not activate the upper rectus abdominis and pull the rib cage forwards, as with sit-ups and "crunches." This movement also results in a simultaneous reflex activation of the back muscles of the lower thoracic spine (the lower thoracic erector spinae).[26,80]

Therefore, whenever sitting, always remember to first gently press back against the sacral support. With practice, you will naturally maintain this pressure and the proper activation of the transversus throughout the sitting period.

The activation of the transversus abdominis muscle when sitting facilitates proper diaphragmatic breathing and causes a beneficial increase in the intra-abdominal

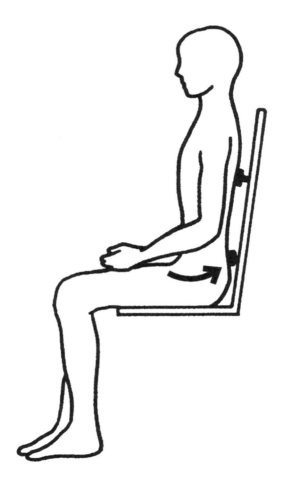

Figure 31.

To activate the lower transversus abdominis muscle when sitting,
press **gently** back against the sacral support in a backward and
upward direction (a backward scooping motion).
IMPORTANT: Do not hold your breath or strain when
practicing this movement.

pressure. The end result is a lengthened spine with decreased compressive stress on the lower back.

Forward-Leaning Posture

When leaning forward from the hips, there is a slight rocking over the sitting bones (the ischial tuberosities) and a tendency for the pelvis to slide backward on the seat.[81] The combination of proper sacral support, along with an open space below the sacral support for the buttocks, results in the ZACKBACK Solution providing proper pelvic and spinal stabilization in a forward-leaning posture (Figure 32).

Crossing the Legs

Why is crossing the legs such a common postural habit when sitting? In most cases, it is a spontaneous attempt to stabilize the body, especially the pelvis.[82] In other words, if certain chair features such as the seat surface and back support fail to properly stabilize the sitter (as usually occurs), then the person must stabilize himself/herself by crossing the legs.[67,83]

However, crossing the legs results in an unhealthy asymmetrical sitting posture. Besides increasing one's sitting fatigue, this posture flexes the lower back and curves the spine sideways.

Another benefit of the ZACKBACK Solution with sacral support is that the pelvis is properly stabilized *without* the need to cross the legs.

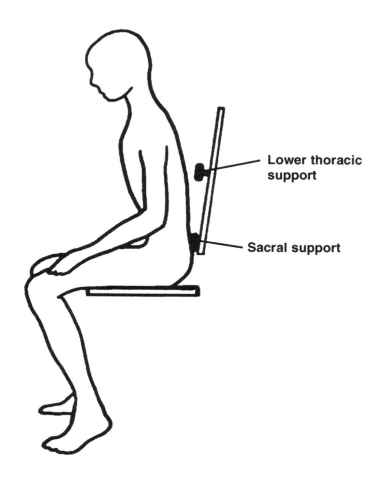

Figure 32.

Proper forward leaning involves bending only at the hips and
keeping your back as straight as possible. When leaning forward,
concentrate on pressing back against the sacral support.

LOWER THORACIC SUPPORT

The key to stabilizing the rib cage is to provide proper support to the lower thoracic spine at the level of the tenth thoracic through the twelfth thoracic vertebrae (T10-T12). This is the only way to correct the main postural fault of sitting, the postural depression or hinging forward of the rib cage towards the pelvis.

Proper lower thoracic support will elevate the rib cage and restore the proper upright relationship of the rib cage and pelvis, bringing the upper trunk over the hips (instead of in front of or behind the hips). In addition, the head, neck, upper back, and shoulders can **only** be brought into proper alignment through lower thoracic support, not through lumbar support or reclining the backrest (Figure 33).

By bringing the head, neck, upper back, and shoulders into proper alignment with lower thoracic support, individuals with pain in the arms, wrists, and hands often notice improvement. In many of these cases, the upper extremity pain is actually originating from the lower neck and upper back (lower cervical and upper thoracic spine).[84-86] These individuals are frequently misdiagnosed as having carpal tunnel syndrome.

Proper Diaphragmatic Breathing

More good news regarding lower thoracic support: Without the need for any exercises, you can immediately experience proper diaphragmatic breathing when sitting, along with a decrease in the stress placed on the scalene

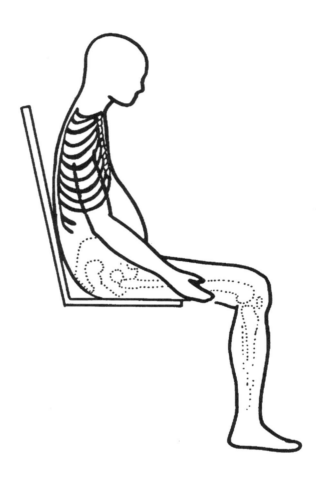

Figure 33-A.

Sitting in a postural depression.

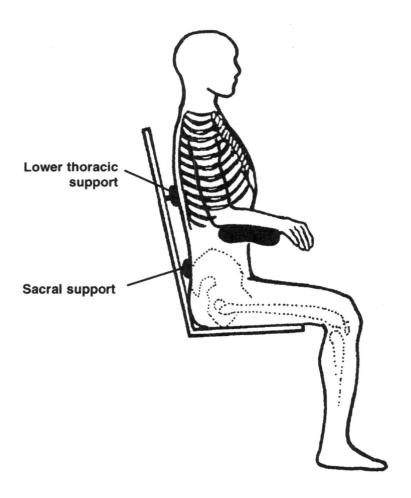

Lower thoracic support

Sacral support

Figure 33-B.

Lower thoracic support will elevate the rib cage and restore
the proper upright relationship of the rib cage and pelvis. Only
lower thoracic support can properly align the head, neck, upper
back, and shoulders.

91

muscles. (Remember, when sitting in a position of postural depression, the scalene muscles are the neck muscles that are overworked in upper chest breathing and in elevating the upper rib cage against gravity.)

Dramatic improvement in diaphragmatic breathing occurs for two reasons:

1. Mechanical support to the lower thoracic spine elevates the rib cage and prevents its downward movement. This mechanical support immediately reduces some of the static load on the scalene muscles.

2. The pressure from the lower thoracic support against the lower thoracic region of the back immediately facilitates proper diaphragmatic breathing by eliciting what are called the intercostal-to-phrenic reflexes.[36,37] In other words, the nerve connected to the diaphragm muscle (the phrenic nerve) is under the control of reflexes that are activated by sensory stimulation of other nerves in the region of the lower thoracic spine. Pressure from the lower thoracic support against this *specific* region of the back is one way to elicit these reflexes.

Thoracic Spinal Mobility

Lower thoracic support also plays an important role in maintaining the ability to fully straighten the thoracic spine. The inability to straighten the thoracic spine is usually associated with old age. However, it has been shown that many individuals can begin to lose this thoracic spinal mobility while still in their twenties, thirties, and forties![87,88]

Location of Lower Thoracic Support

To find the proper location for lower thoracic support, you will need the assistance of another person.

While sitting in an upright, relaxed posture with sacral support in position and hands in the lap, have your assistant locate the lower tips of your shoulder blades (scapulae) (Figure 34). With your assistant's thumbs on your spine at the level of your armpits, have your assistant slide the thumbs directly sideways in opposite directions until he/she feels the inner edges of your shoulder blades. The lower tips of the shoulder blades will be located at the bottom of the inner edges of the shoulder blades. Have your assistant slide the thumbs down the inner edges of your shoulder blades until he/she comes to the lower tips of your shoulder blades.

The upper border of the thoracic support should be positioned from 1 inch to approximately 3 inches below the lower tips of your shoulder blades. To find the exact location for the lower thoracic support within this range, have your assistant stand at your left side and stabilize your trunk by placing his/her left hand on your right shoulder. Then have your assistant gently press the palm of his/her right hand against your lower thoracic spine, starting at 1 inch below the lower tips of your shoulder blades.

Your assistant should continue to gently press into your back while lowering the palm about ¼ inch at a time, until the palm is approximately 3 inches below the lower tips of your shoulder blades.

You are trying to find the position for support that results in the most dramatic elevation of your rib cage,

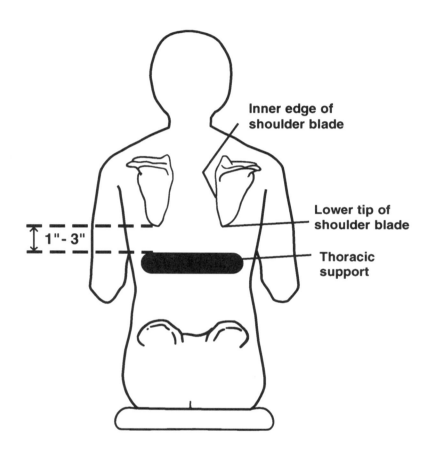

**Inner edge of
shoulder blade**

**Lower tip of
shoulder blade**

**Thoracic
support**

1" - 3"

Figure 34.
Proper location of lower thoracic support.
IMPORTANT: The most common mistake is to have the thoracic
support positioned too high (too close to the shoulder blades). The
upper border of the thoracic support needs to be *at least one inch
below* the lower tips of the shoulder blades.

without pushing your head and shoulders slightly forward (support is too high) or causing your upper trunk to arch backward (support is too low). The correct position should feel the most comfortable. You may also experience an immediate improvement in your breathing, along with less tension in your neck and upper back.

As a mock-up lower thoracic support, attach to your chair in the proper location using VELCRO® or tape, a firm piece of foam approximately 4 inches in height, 10 inches wide, and 1 to 3 inches thick.

The thickness of the thoracic support you require will depend on the mobility of your thoracic spine and the angle of recline of your chair's backrest. Optimal healthy upright posture is not exactly vertical. In order to balance your trunk, you will only lean back approximately 3 to 5 degrees from fully vertical. (See Figure 33-B.) With the proper balanced posture, you should easily be able to maintain gentle pressure against both the thoracic and sacral supports.

If the thoracic support is too thick, you will feel that you are being pushed forward off balance, or you will start to lose contact with the sacral support. If the thoracic support is too thin, you will have to arch your trunk backward in order to contact it.

> **Important Note:** A lower thoracic support is contraindicated for those individuals with a rigid round back (called a fixed thoracic kyphosis). In these individuals, the lower thoracic support will just push the trunk forward without elevating the rib cage.

ZACKBACK DYNAMIC SITTING

According to a July 21, 1997 *Wall Street Journal* article,[89] the new sitting solution from the office furniture industry is now "active sitting" on chairs that promote continuous movement. Unfortunately, the office furniture industry's approach to active (dynamic) sitting reflects a total misunderstanding of the functioning of the human body.

The human body can be compared to an open-chain system of links that allows free movement at the various joints.[82] Sitting, however, involves a spontaneous attempt to *stabilize* the body segments.[67] This need for stability demands a closed-chain system of links[90] (Figure 35).

The healthiest and most efficient closed-chain link system for sitting is stabilization of the trunk through proper activation of the diaphragm, transversus abdominis, and the back muscles of the lower thoracic spine. *This is the basis for ZACKBACK Sitting and true dynamic sitting posture.*

Proper trunk stabilization allows free, efficient movement of the arms without the need for arm support. (The proper seat height, seat depth, and rounded front edge to the seat allow important leg position changes.[15,91])

Continuous movement on a chair while sitting in the typical position of postural depression is *not* promoting proper dynamic sitting. Instead, it is simply promoting the postural breakdown of the body while moving.

Health professionals advocating continuous movement when sitting always refer to the beneficial effect this movement will have on the discs of the spine.

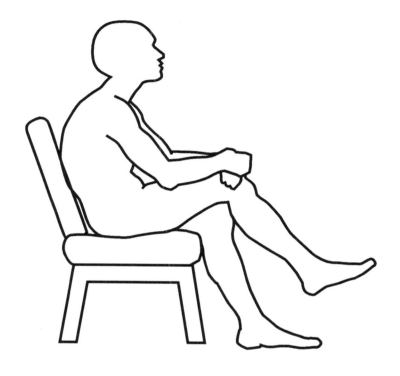

Figure 35.

A typical closed-chain position to stabilize the body
segments when sitting.

However, a greater health benefit to the spinal discs occurs by walking during breaks from sitting, and also by walking as a daily aerobic exercise.[92,93]

Fidgeting

Fidgeting when sitting should not be considered healthy. It is actually a sensitive indicator of postural stress and discomfort.[94,95]

Two of the main causes of fidgeting are:

1. The unbalancing of the body caused by the design of chair backrests.[96,97] When leaning against the typical chair backrest, the center of gravity of the trunk is displaced behind the pelvis. This distorts the proper upright relationship of the head, neck, rib cage, and pelvis, and it leads to fatigue and fidgeting.

2. Impaired respiration (poor diaphragmatic breathing) from sitting in a position of postural depression. In 1896, Kellogg[98] described the individual breathing in a slumped sitting position as being "constantly in a state of air starvation, a fact which is evidenced by the disposition to straighten up and draw a long, deep breath every now and then, which is constantly noticed in persons who habitually sit... in a stooped attitude."

By promoting proper diaphragmatic breathing and the proper upright relationship of the head, neck, rib cage, and pelvis, ZACKBACK Sitting greatly reduces fatigue and fidgeting. Through the postural re-education of ZACKBACK Sitting, one quickly becomes very sensitive to the postural distortion induced by chairs with reclining backrests, lumbar supports, and support to the upper back and shoulder blades.

ZACKBACK SITTING AT THE COMPUTER WORKSTATION

When adjusting the computer workstation, the first consideration should always be achieving your optimal healthy sitting posture with proper sacral and lower thoracic support. Next, address arm and hand posture by deciding on the best position for the keyboard and mouse. Finally, address head posture and the visual demands of the task by deciding on the best location for the computer screen and documents.[99]

FINDING THE IDEAL CHAIR

It is important to realize that the mock-up approach just described using sacral and lower thoracic foam pads is a low-end solution that only *minimally* approaches the dramatic results of the ZACKBACK Solution.

Over the 10 years since I first developed the ZACKBACK Solution, I have found the only way to dramatically relieve low back pain, upper back pain, neck pain, carpal tunnel syndrome, and dramatically improve both sitting posture and standing posture is with a specialized, fully adjustable chair that addresses all of the following issues:

- Sacral support of the proper shape, firmness, and dimensions that is adjustable in height, depth, and angle.

- Lower thoracic support of the proper shape, firmness, and dimensions that is adjustable in height and depth.
- Proper angle to the backrest.
- Proper slope to the seat to facilitate pelvic and spinal stabilization.
- Proper contouring of the seat and friction of the seat fabric for pelvic and spinal stabilization.
- Proper seat cushioning to stabilize the pelvis and prevent weight bearing on the tail bone and trochanters.
- Proper seat height adjustment range to allow the feet to be placed firmly on the floor.
- Proper location of the armrests on the chair to prevent collapsing the body weight forward on the armrests.

Just as important with such a specialized, fully adjustable chair are **key areas that should not be supported.** These areas are:

1. The posterior buttocks.

An open space is necessary below the sacral support for the posterior protrusion of the buttocks. Without such an open space, the buttocks will be pushed forwards on the seat, inhibiting proper pelvic and spinal stabilization.[100]

2. The lumbar spine.

By adding lumbar support, one drastically alters the ZACKBACK Solution. The proper upright relationship of the rib cage and pelvis is altered, with the upper trunk being displaced behind the hips. There is also a spontaneous relaxation of the abdominal muscles.

3. The upper back and shoulder blades.

Any back support above the lower thoracic spine is detrimental to healthy sitting posture by pushing the head and shoulders forward, and inhibiting proper diaphragmatic breathing.[15,101-103]

My research on chair designs has found that no chair on the market comes close to even minimally employing the ZACKBACK Solution. Moreover, most chair designs on the market actually *inhibit* the ZACKBACK Solution!

Therefore, I have spent the last 10 years developing what I consider to be the optimal solution to healthy, pain-free sitting — the patented ZACKBACK® Posture Chair (Figure 36).

Since August 1993, the State of Minnesota, Department of Administration has conducted sitting trials with its employees using the ZACKBACK Posture Chair.[104] The sitting trials have lasted from a minimum of one week to over four years in some cases.

Through October 1997, 152 employees have evaluated the ZACKBACK Posture Chair, and 88.2% of these individuals reported that the ZACKBACK Posture Chair either eliminated or reduced their pain, increased their comfort, or improved their posture. **These results are even more impressive considering that the vast majority of these individuals were using state of the art ergonomic chairs before trying the ZACKBACK Posture Chair!** These ergonomic chairs had features including lumbar support, reclining backrests, forward-sloping seat adjustments, and adjustable armrests.

ZACKBACK CHAIR FEATURES (See Figure 36)

1. **Sacral support adjusts in height, depth, and angle** - critical for stabilizing the pelvis in its proper neutral position. Also stabilizes the lumbar spine and sacroiliac joints.

2. **Lower thoracic support adjusts in height and depth** - critical for proper alignment of the trunk, shoulder girdle, head, and neck. Stabilizes the rib cage, prevents slumped posture, and promotes proper diaphragmatic breathing.

3. **No support to upper back and shoulder blades** - detrimental to healthy sitting posture by pushing the shoulders and head forward, and inhibiting diaphragmatic breathing.

4. **No lumbar support** - detrimental to healthy sitting posture by distorting the proper upright relationship of the rib cage and pelvis, with the upper trunk being displaced behind the hips. Sitting with lumbar support will relax the lower abdominal muscles and increase stress to the neck and upper back.

5. **No support to the posterior buttocks** - detrimental to healthy sitting posture by pushing the buttocks forward on the seat, and preventing proper pelvic and spinal stabilization.

6. **Armrests adjust in height, width, depth, and can be rotated inwards and outwards** - are positioned on chair to facilitate use of backrest and to prevent collapsing body weight forward on the armrests.

7. **Firm, contoured seat** - facilitates use of backrest, stabilizes the pelvis, and prevents weight bearing on the tail bone.

8. **Pneumatic, adjustable seat height** - critical for proper sitting stability with the feet firmly on the floor.

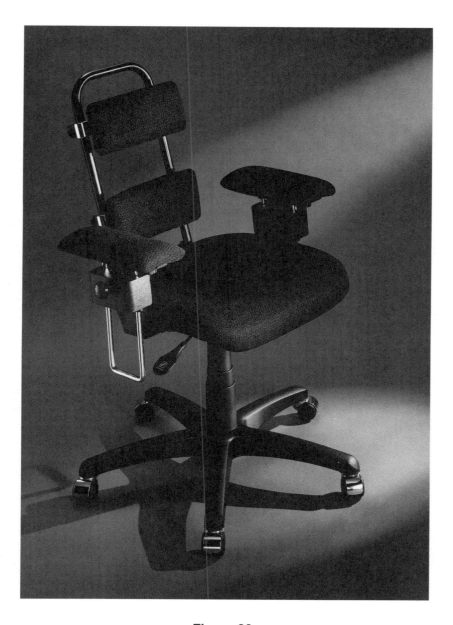

Figure 36.

The patented ZACKBACK® Posture Chair, invented by
Dennis Zacharkow, PT.

A further breakdown of the results through October 1997 of this ongoing study is as follows:

The ZACKBACK Posture Chair...
- Eliminated or reduced pain — 50.7%
- Increased Comfort— 26.3%
- Improved Posture — 11.2%
- Was uncomfortable — 9.2%
- Increased pain — 0.7%
- No opinion or not sure — 1.9%

NOTE: This data is based on the primary comment of the 152 individuals evaluating the ZACKBACK Posture Chair.

Regarding specific results for pain relief, 98 of the 152 individuals reported pain at the start of the ZACKBACK sitting trials when sitting in other ergonomic chairs. **The ZACKBACK Posture Chair eliminated or reduced pain in 78.6% of these individuals!** Areas of pain relief included the lower back, mid-back, upper back, neck, shoulders, arms, wrists, and hands.

The dramatic results achieved by the ZACKBACK Posture Chair in pain relief and posture improvement have been very gratifying to me. Unfortunately, my chair is advocated by very few doctors, physical therapists, and chiropractors, because the ZACKBACK Solution contradicts their established treatment programs. Imagine the money that could be saved if these health professionals recommended the ZACKBACK Posture Chair at the initial evaluation or early on in the treatment program!

With the ZACKBACK Posture Chair there is a guarantee: ZACKBACK is guaranteed to *relieve* your pain and *improve* your posture. If it does not, just call my company within 30 days after receiving your chair and return it for a full refund. You won't find a better guarantee anywhere for relieving your pain! (If you are currently being treated by a doctor, physical therapist, or chiropractor, try asking for the same guarantee.)

I hope my book has made you aware of the importance of healthy sitting posture and also enlightened you regarding long-standing sitting misconceptions. If you sit in a chair all day long and experience pain and fatigue, I hope you will give the ZACKBACK Solution a try. You have nothing to lose except your pain.

REFERENCES

1. *Consumer Reports*, 61:26, September 1996.

2. Dagostino, M.: Lumbar support most critical feature to consider during chair selection. *Occupational Health and Safety*, 63:63-65, March 1994.

3. Pierson, J.: Stand up and listen: your chair may harm your health. *The Wall Street Journal*, September 12, 1995, pp. B-1, B-10.

4. Grant, C.: Built to last: Your body and the ergonomically correct workspace. *Safe Workplace*, 5:14-16, Winter 1997.

5. Anderson, T. McC.: *Human Kinetics and Analysing Body Movements.* London, Heinemann, 1951.

6. Alexander, F.M.: *Man's Supreme Inheritance.* New York, Dutton, 1918.

7. Cohen, L.A.: Role of eye and neck proprioceptive mechanisms in body orientation and motor coordination. *Journal of Neurophysiology*, 24:1-11, 1961.

8. Laville, A.: Postural stress in high-speed precision work. *Ergonomics*, 28:229-236, 1985.

9. Paris, S.V.: Cervical symptoms of forward head posture. *Topics in Geriatric Rehabilitation*, 5(4):11-19, 1990.

10. Stewart, S.F.: Physiology of the unshod and shod foot with an evolutionary history of footgear. *American Journal of Surgery*, 68:127-138, 1945.

11. Leibowitz, J.: For the victims of our culture: the Alexander technique. *Dance Scope*, 4:32-37, 1967.

12. Åkerblom, B.: *Standing and Sitting Posture.* Stockholm, Nordiska Bokhandeln, 1948.

13. Andersson, G.B.J., Murphy, R.W., Örtengren, R., and Nachemson, A.L.: The influence of backrest inclination and lumbar support on lumbar lordosis. *Spine*, 4:52-58, 1979.

14. Bridger, R.S., Wilkinson, D., and Van Houweninge, T.: Hip joint mobility and spinal angles in standing and in different sitting postures. *Human Factors*, 31:229-241, 1989.

15. Zacharkow, D.: *Posture: Sitting, Standing, Chair Design and Exercise.* Springfield, Thomas, 1988.

16. Zacharkow, D.: The problems with lumbar support. *Physical Therapy Forum*, 9(35):1,3-5, 1990.

17. Branton, P.: Behaviour, body mechanics and discomfort. In Grandjean, E. (Ed.): *Proceedings of the Symposium on Sitting Posture.* London, Taylor and Francis, 1969, pp. 202-213.

18. Sandover, J., and Dupuis, H.: A reanalysis of spinal motion during vibration. *Ergonomics*, 30:975-985, 1987.

19. McKenzie, R.A.: *The Lumbar Spine. Mechanical Diagnosis and Therapy.* Waikanae, Spinal Publications, 1981.

20. Humphry, G.M.: *A Treatise on the Human Skeleton.* Cambridge, MacMillan, 1858.

21. Wiles, P.: Postural deformities of the anteroposterior curves of the spine. *The Lancet*, 1:911-919, April 17, 1937.

22. Vulcan, A.P., King, A.I., and Nakamura, G.S.: Effects of bending on the vertebral column during $+G_z$ acceleration. *Aerospace Medicine*, 41:294-300, 1970.

23. Alexander, C.J.: Scheuermann's disease. *Skeletal Radiology*, 1:209-221, 1977.

24. Markolf, K.L.: Deformation of the thoracolumbar intervertebral joints in response to external loads. *The Journal of Bone and Joint Surgery*, 54-A:511-533, 1972.

25. White, A.A., and Panjabi, M.M.: *Clinical Biomechanics of the Spine.* Philadelphia, Lippincott, 1978, p.84.

26. Haynes, R.S.: Postural reflexes. *American Journal of Diseases of Children*, 36:1093-1107, 1928.

27. De Troyer, A.: Mechanical role of the abdominal muscles in relation to posture. *Respiration Physiology*, 53:341-353, 1983.

28. Watson, P.J., and Hixon, T.J.: Respiratory kinematics in classical (opera) singers. *Journal of Speech and Hearing Research*, 28:104-122, 1985.

29. Xie, A., Takasaki, Y., Popkin, J., Orr, D., and Bradley, T.D.: Chemical and postural influence on scalene and diaphragmatic activation in humans. *Journal of Applied Physiology*, 70:658-664, 1991.

30. Xie, A., Takasaki, Y., and Bradley, T.D.: Influence of body position on diaphragmatic and scalene activation during hypoxic rebreathing. *Journal of Applied Physiology*, 75:2234-2238, 1993.

31. Travell, J.G., and Simons, D.G.: *Myofascial Pain and Dysfunction*. Baltimore, Williams and Wilkins, 1983.

32. Narakas, A.O.: The role of thoracic outlet syndrome in the double crush syndrome. *Annals of Hand and Upper Limb Surgery*, 9:331-340, 1990.

33. Novak, C.B., Mackinnon, S.E., and Patterson, G.A.: Evaluation of patients with thoracic outlet syndrome. *The Journal of Hand Surgery*, 18A:292-299, 1993.

34. Mackinnon, S.E., and Novak, C.B.: Clinical commentary: pathogenesis of cumulative trauma disorder. *The Journal of Hand Surgery*, 19A:873-883, 1994.

35. Zacharkow, D.: Sitting posture: the overlooked factor in carpal tunnel syndrome. *Advance for Physical Therapists*, 5:8-9, 17, May 16, 1994.

36. Decima, E.E., von Euler, C., and Thoden, U.: Intercostal-to-phrenic reflexes in the spinal cat. *Acta Physiologica Scandinavica*, 75:568-579, 1969.

37. Leanderson, R., Sundberg, J., and von Euler, C.: Role of diaphragmatic activity during singing: a study of transdiaphragmatic pressures. *Journal of Applied Physiology*, 62:259-270, 1987.

38. Sarti, M.A., Monfort, M., Fuster, M.A., and Villaplana, L.A.: Muscle activity in upper and lower rectus abdominis during abdominal exercises. *Archives of Physical Medicine and Rehabilitation*, 77:1293-1297, 1996.

39. Floyd, W.F., and Silver, P.H.S.: Electromyographic study of patterns of activity of the anterior abdominal wall muscles in man. *Journal of Anatomy*, 84:132-145, 1950.

40. Lipetz, S., and Gutin, B.: An electromyographic study of four abdominal exercises. *Medicine and Science in Sports*, 2:35-38, 1970.

41. Frost, L.H.: Individual structural differences in the orthopedic examination. *Journal of Health and Physical Education*, 9:90-93,122, 1938.

42. Drew, L.C.: *Individual Gymnastics*, 5th ed. Philadelphia, Lea and Febiger, 1945.

43. De Troyer, A., Estenne, M., Ninane, V., Van Gansbeke, D., and Gorini M.: Transversus abdominis muscle function in humans. *Journal of Applied Physiology*, 68:1010-1016, 1990.

44. Cresswell, A.G., Grundström, H., and Thorstensson, A.: Observations on intra-abdominal pressure and patterns of abdominal intra-muscular activity in man. *Acta Physiologica Scandinavica*, 144:409-418, 1992.

45. Ono, K.: Electromyographic studies of the abdominal wall muscles in visceroptosis. *The Tohoku Journal of Experimental Medicine*, 68:347-354, 1958.

46. Hodges, P.W., and Richardson, C.A.: Inefficient muscular stabilization of the lumbar spine associated with low back pain. *Spine*, 21:2640-2650, 1996.

47. Keith, A.: Man's posture: its evolution and disorders. Lecture four. The adaptations of the abdomen and of its viscera to the orthograde posture. *The British Medical Journal*, 1:587-590, 1923.

48. Parsons, C.A.: Use of wrist rests by data input VDU operators. In Lovesey, E.J. (Ed.): *Contemporary Ergonomics*. London, Taylor and Francis, 1991, pp.319-322.

49. Pascarelli, E.P., and Kella, J.J.: Soft-tissue injuries related to use of the computer keyboard. *Journal of Occupational Medicine*, 35:522-532, 1993.

50. Harvey, R., and Peper, E.: Surface electromyography and mouse use position. *Ergonomics*, 40:781-789, 1997.

51. Straker, L.M., Pollock, C.M., and Mangharam, J.E.: The effect of shoulder posture on performance, discomfort and muscle fatigue whilst working on a visual display unit. *International Journal of Industrial Ergonomics*, 20:1-10, 1997.

52. Mosher, E.M.: The influence of habitual posture on the symmetry and health of the body. *The Brooklyn Medical Journal*, 6:393-414, 1892.

110

53. Avon, G., and Schmitt, L.: Electromyographie du trapèze dans diverses positions de travail à la machine à écrire. *Ergonomics*, 18:619-626, 1975.

54. Stack, B.: *Keyboard RSI: The Practical Solution.* Hobart, Tasmania, Muden Publishing Company, 1987.

55. Werner, R., Armstrong, T.J., Bir, C., and Aylard, M.K.: Intracarpal canal pressures: the role of finger, hand, wrist and forearm position. *Clinical Biomechanics*, 12:44-51, 1997.

56. Pechan, J., and Julis, I.: The pressure measurement in the ulnar nerve. A contribution to the pathophysiology of the cubital tunnel syndrome. *Journal of Biomechanics*, 8:75-79, 1975.

57. Hedge, A., and Powers, J.R.: Wrist postures while keyboarding: effects of a negative slope keyboard system and full motion forearm supports. *Ergonomics*, 38:508-517, 1995.

58. DiVeta, J., Walker, M.L., and Skibinski, B.: Relationship between performance of selected scapular muscles and scapular abduction in standing subjects. *Physical Therapy*, 70:470-479, 1990.

59. Lovett, R.W.: Round shoulders and faulty attitude: a method of observation and record, with conclusions as to treatment. *Boston Medical and Surgical Journal*, 147:510-520, 1902.

60. Fahrner: *Das Kind und der Schultisch.* Zurich, Schulthess, 1865. Translated in Cohn, H.: *The Hygiene of the Eye in Schools.* London, Simpkin, Marshall and Co., 1886, pp. 94-98.

61. Sucher, B.M., and Heath, D.M.: Thoracic outlet syndrome—a myofascial variant: part three. Structural and postural considerations. *The Journal of the American Osteopathic Association*, 93:334, 340-345, 1993.

62. Sucher, B.M.: Thoracic outlet syndrome — a myofascial variant: part one. Pathology and diagnosis. *The Journal of the American Osteopathic Association*, 90:686-704, 1990.

63. Fleischer, A.G., Rademacher, U., and Windberg, H.J.: Individual characteristics of sitting behaviour. *Ergonomics*, 30:703-709, 1987.

64. Forssberg, H., and Hirschfeld, H.: Postural adjustments in sitting humans following external perturbations: muscle activity and kinematics. *Experimental Brain Research*, 97:515-527, 1994.

65. Bennett, H.E.: *School Posture and Seating.* Boston, Ginn and Company, 1928.

66. Helbig, K.: Sitzdruckverteilung beim ungepolsterten sitz. *Anthropologischer Anzieger,* 36:194-202, 1978.

67. Branton, P.: *The Comfort of Easy Chairs.* Stevenage, Hertfordshire, England, The Furniture Industry Research Association, 1966.

68. Bendix, T., Winkel, J., and Jessen, F.: Comparison of office chairs with fixed forwards or backwards inclining, or tiltable seats. *European Journal of Applied Physiology,* 54:378-385, 1985.

69. Freudenthal, A., van Riel, M.P.J.M., Molenbroek, J.F.M., and Snijders, C.J.: The effect on sitting posture of a desk with a ten-degree inclination using an adjustable chair and table. *Applied Ergonomics,* 22:329-336, 1991.

70. Jaschinski-Kruza, W.: Visual strain during VDU work: the effect of viewing distance and dark focus. *Ergonomics,* 31:1449-1465, 1988.

71. Grandjean, E.: Postures and the design of VDT workstations. *Behaviour and Information Technology,* 3:301-311, 1984.

72. Jaschinski-Kruza, W.: Eyestrain in VDU users: viewing distance and the resting position of ocular muscles. *Human Factors,* 33:69-83, 1991.

73. Jaschinski-Kruza, W.: On the preferred viewing distances to screen and document at VDU workplaces. *Ergonomics,* 33:1055-1063, 1990.

74. Coe, J.B.: The posture factor in repetitive stain injuries. In *Ergonomics in New Zealand. Proceedings of the Inaugural Conference of the New Zealand Ergonomics Society.* Palmerston North, New Zealand Ergonomics Society, 1987, pp. 114-124.

75. Sheedy, J.E., and Parsons, S.D.: Vision and the video display terminal: clinical findings. In Sauter, S., Dainoff, M., and Smith, M. (Eds.): *Promoting Health and Productivity in the Computerized Office.* London, Taylor and Francis, 1990, pp. 197-206.

76. Martin, D.K., and Dain, S.J.: Postural modifications of VDU operators wearing bifocal spectacles. *Applied Ergonomics,* 19:293-300, 1988.

112

77. Goldman, J.M., Lehr, R.P., Millar, A.B., and Silver, J.R.: An electromyographic study of the abdominal muscles during postural and respiratory manoeuvres. *Journal of Neurology, Neurosurgery, and Psychiatry,* 50:866-869, 1987.

78. Strohl, K.P., Mead, J., Banzett, R.B., Loring, S.H., and Kosch, P.C.: Regional differences in abdominal muscle activity during various maneuvers in humans. *Journal of Applied Physiology,* 51:1471-1476, 1981.

79. O'Sullivan, P.B., Twomey, L., Allison, G.T., Sinclair, J., Miller, K., and Knox, J.: Altered patterns of abdominal muscle activation in patients with chronic low back pain. *Australian Journal of Physiotherapy,* 43:91-98, 1997.

80. Rathbone, J.L., and Hunt, V.V.: *Corrective Physical Education,* 7th ed. Philadelphia, Saunders, 1965.

81. Cotton, F.J.: School furniture for Boston schools. *American Physical Education Review,* 9:267-284, 1904.

82. Dempster, W.T.: The anthropometry of body action. *Annals of the New York Academy of Sciences,* 63:559-585, 1955.

83. Branton, P., and Grayson, G.: An evaluation of train seats by observation of sitting behaviour. *Ergonomics,* 10:35-51, 1967.

84. Wong, E., Lee, G., Zucherman, J., and Mason, D.T.: Successful management of female office workers with "repetitive stress injury" or "carpal tunnel syndrome" by a new treatment modality — application of low level laser. *International Journal of Clinical Pharmacology and Therapeutics,* 33:208-211, 1995.

85. Farfan, H.F., and Baldwin, J.: Tired neck syndrome: chronic postural strain. In Karwowski, W. (Ed.): *Trends in Ergonomics/Human Factors III.* Amsterdam, Elsevier Science, 1986, pp. 651-658.

86. Harms-Ringdahl, K., and Ekholm, J.: Intensity and character of pain and muscular activity levels elicited by maintained extreme flexion position of the lower-cervical-upper-thoracic spine. *Scandinavian Journal of Rehabilitation Medicine,* 18:117-126, 1986.

87. O'Gorman, H., and Jull, G.: Thoracic kyphosis and mobility: the effect of age. *Physiotherapy Practice,* 3:154-162, 1987.

88. Cutler, W.B., Friedmann, E., and Genovese-Stone, E.: Prevalence of kyphosis in a healthy sample of pre- and postmenopausal

women. *American Journal of Physical Medicine and Rehabilitation*, 72:219-225, 1993.

89. Takahashi, C.: Office chair encourages "active sitting." *The Wall Street Journal*, July 21, 1997, pp. B-1, B-10.

90. Evans, E.: Ergonomic aspects of the driving position—a postural analysis. In *Ergonomics in the Tourist, Agricultural and Mining Industries. Proceedings of the 22nd Annual Conference of the Ergonomics Society of Australia and New Zealand*. Carlton South, Victoria, Australia, ESANZ, 1985, pp. 250-255.

91. Keegan, J.J.: Alterations of the lumbar curve related to posture and seating. *The Journal of Bone and Joint Surgery*, 35-A:589-603, 1953.

92. Holm, S., and Nachemson, A.: Variations in the nutrition of the canine intervertebral disc induced by motion. *Spine*, 8:866-874, 1983.

93. Helander, M.G., and Quance, L.A.: Effect of work-rest schedules on spinal shrinkage in the sedentary worker. *Applied Ergonomics*, 21:279-284, 1990.

94. Bhatnager, V., Drury, C.G., and Schiro, S.G.: Posture, postural discomfort, and performance. *Human Factors*, 27:189-199, 1985.

95. Grandjean, E., Jenni, M., and Rhiner, A.: Eine indirekte methode zur erfassung des komfortgefühls beim sitzen. *Internationale Zeitschrift für Angewandte Physiologie Einschliesslich Arbeitsphysiologie*, 18: 101-106, 1960.

96. Mosher, E.M.: Hygienic desks for school children. *Educational Review*, 18:9-14, 1899.

97. Stewart, P.C., and McQuilton, G.: Straddle seating for the cerebral palsied child. *Physiotherapy*, 73:204-206, 1987.

98. Kellogg, J.H.: Physical deterioration resulting from school life; cause; remedy. *Proceedings of the National Education Association*, 1896, pp. 899-911.

99. Darby, F.W.: *Visual Display Unit Operators: A Study of Their Postures and Workstations.* Department of Health, Southern Regional Occupational Health Unit, Wellington, New Zealand, 1984.

100. Taylor, H.L.: Results of research on conditions affecting posture. *Journal of the American Medical Association*, 68:327-330, 1917.

114

101. Romaniuk, J.R., Supinski, G.S., and DiMarco, A.F.: Reflex control of diaphragm activation by thoracic afferents. *Journal of Applied Physiology*, 75:63-69, 1993.

102. Remmers, J.E.: Extra-segmental reflexes derived from intercostal afferents: phrenic and laryngeal responses. *Journal of Physiology*, 233:45-62, 1973.

103. Branton, P.: Backshapes of seated persons — how close can the interface be designed? *Applied Ergonomics*, 15:105-107, 1984.

104. Study conducted by Stephen C. Hendrickson, M.S., Safety Director and Workers' Compensation Coordinator, State of Minnesota, Department of Administration, 50 Sherburne Avenue, 114 Administration Building, St. Paul, MN 55155, August 1993-October 1997.

RESOURCES

ZACKBACK® POSTURE CHAIR

For information on the ZACKBACK Posture Chair
Phone: 1-800-SITTING
Write: ZACKBACK International, Inc.
PO Box 9100
Rochester, MN 55903
Website: www.zackback.com
e-mail: zmail@zackback.com

READING STANDS / DOCUMENT HOLDERS

- The **Atlas**™ is a reading stand/document holder that is adjustable in both height and angle.
  Phone: 1-800-GET-ATLAS
  Write: Dainoff Designs, Inc.
  8606 Empire Court
  Cincinnati, OH 45231-4913

- Various designs of reading stands are available from the LEVENGER® catalog.
  Phone: 1-800-544-0880
  Write: LEVENGER
  420 South Congress Avenue
  Delray Beach, FL 33445-4696

DOWNWARD-SLOPING KEYBOARD TRAYS

• Several adjustable models are available from
WORKRITE® Ergonomics.
Phone: 415-884-2311
Write: WORKRITE Ergonomics
77 Digital Drive
Novato, CA 94949

TECHNICAL PAPERS

If you plan on discussing the ZACKBACK Solution with your M.D., physical therapist, chiropractor, or other health professional, the following technical papers by Dennis Zacharkow, PT are available upon request:

• *The Problems with Lumbar Support*

• *Sitting Posture: The Overlooked Factor in Carpal Tunnel Syndrome*

(The above technical papers are also available on the ZACKBACK website at www.zackback.com)

INDEX

ZACKBACK SITTING
Phone/Fax/Mail Order Form

Phone orders: **Call Toll Free 1-800-SITTING**
(or 507-252-9293)
Fax orders: **507-252-5150**

Mail orders: **ZACKBACK International, Inc.**
P.O. Box 9100
Rochester, MN 55903

Please send _____ copy (ies) of ZACKBACK SITTING
by Dennis Zacharkow, PT
Price: **$13.95** (U.S.)
Sales Tax: Please add 6.5% (90¢ per book) to books
shipped to Minnesota addresses
Shipping & Packing: **$3.00** for the first book.
Add **$1.00** for each additional book.

Ship to:

Name_____

Address_____

City_____ State_____ Zip _____

Phone _____

PAYMENT METHOD:

☐ Check or money order enclosed payable to
ZACKBACK International, Inc.

☐ VISA   ☐ MasterCard

Account No.
☐☐☐☐ ☐☐☐☐ ☐☐☐☐ ☐☐☐☐

Exp. Date
☐☐ ☐☐

Month Year   Signature (required for credit card orders)

**The ZACKBACK
Guarantee:**

ZACKBACK
International, Inc. is con-
fident you will find this
unique book to be worth
far more than your pur-
chase price. If for any
reason you do not agree,
we will promptly refund
your money.

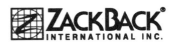

Please inquire regarding volume discounts.
Call Toll Free 1-800-SITTING

ZACKBACK SITTING
Phone/Fax/Mail Order Form

Phone orders: **Call Toll Free 1-800-SITTING**
(or 507-252-9293)
Fax orders: **507-252-5150**

Mail orders: **ZACKBACK International, Inc.**
P.O. Box 9100
Rochester, MN 55903

Please send _____ **copy (ies) of ZACKBACK SITTING**
by Dennis Zacharkow, PT
Price: **$13.95** (U.S.)
Sales Tax: Please add 6.5% (90¢ per book) to books
shipped to Minnesota addresses
Shipping & Packing: **$3.00** for the first book.
Add **$1.00** for each additional book.
Ship to:

Name_____

Address_____

City _____ State_____ Zip _____

Phone _____

PAYMENT METHOD:

☐ Check or money order enclosed payable to
ZACKBACK International, Inc.

☐ VISA   ☐ MasterCard

Account No.
☐☐☐☐ ☐☐☐☐ ☐☐☐☐ ☐☐☐☐

Exp. Date
☐☐ ☐☐

Month   Year

Signature (required for credit card orders)

**The ZACKBACK
Guarantee:**

ZACKBACK
International, Inc. is con-
fident you will find this
unique book to be worth
far more than your pur-
chase price. If for any
reason you do not agree,
we will promptly refund
your money.

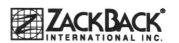

Please inquire regarding volume discounts.
Call Toll Free 1-800-SITTING